Keto Diet Recipes 2021

Delicious and Satiating Recipes to Getting Back In Shape and Burn Fat Fast Effortlessly

Jane Leaner

Please note the information contained within this document is for educational and entertainment purposes only. All effort has been executed to present accurate, up to date, and reliable, complete information. No warranties of any kind are declared or implied. Readers acknowledge that the author is not engaging in the rendering of legal, financial, medical, or professional advice. The content within this book has been derived from various sources. Please consult a licensed professional before attempting any techniques outlined in this book.

By reading this document, the reader agrees that under no circumstances is the author responsible for any losses, direct or indirect, which are incurred as a result of the use of the information contained within this document, including, but not limited to, - errors, omissions, or inaccuracies.

Table of Content

1. Parmesan Beef Slices.. 8
2. Sloppy Ground Beef Joes 10
3. Spinach Beef Heart... 13
4. Taco Tasty Bowls.. 15
5. Quick and Easy Mongolian Beef.. 16
6. Rich Chocolate Mousse 19
7. Smooth Peanut Butter Cream 21
8. Vanilla Avocado Popsicles 22
9. Vanilla Bean Frappuccino.. 23
10. Vegan Pumpkin Pie Chia Pudding 24
11. Yogurt Mint 25
12. Cod Poblano Cream Sauce 27
13. Coleslaw worth a Second Helping 28
14. Fennel and Arugula Salad with Fig Vinaigrette........................... 29
15. Garlic Vinaigrette 31
16. Greek Salad 33
17. Green Beans 35
18. Healthy Broccoli Salad... 37
19. Kohlrabi Cilantro slaw 38
20. Lemon Caper Pesto 39
21. Lemon Kale Cider Vinegar 40
22. Lime Cilantro crema 41
23. Mozzarella Radish Salad 43
24. Mediterranean Chicken Salad 46
25. Mini Zucchini Bites 48
26. Nicoise Salad 49
27. Parsley Pesto 51
28. Pico de Gallo Salad... 52
29. Portobello Italiano Sausage 53
30. Quinoa with Vegetables... 54
31. Romaine Lettuce and Radicchios Mix.. 55
32. Rosemary Creamy Fauxtatoes... 56
33. Shrimp Cobb Salad 58
34. Stewed Herbed Fruit.. 60

35. Stuffed Eggplant Provencale 62
36. Stuffed Mushrooms Feta 65
37. Taste of Normandy Salad 66
38. Tenderloins Mushrooms 69
39. Teriyaki Sauce 71
40. Tomatoes Creamy Garlic Sauce 72
41. Turmeric & Lemon Dressing 73
42. Tzatziki Salad 75
43. Walnut & Mint Pesto 76
44. Walnut Vinaigrette 77
45. Asparagus Avocado Soup 79
46. Buffalo Chicken Soup 82
47. Cheeseburger Soup 85
48. Chicken Enchilada Soup 88
49. Crackpot Chicken Taco Soup 91
50. Creamy Cauliflower Soup 94
51. Cream of Thyme Tomato Soup 97
52. Easy Cauliflower Soup 99
53. Healthy Chicken Taco Soup 101
54. Lime-Mint Soup 103
55. Quick Lentil Chili 104
56. Roasted Tomato Soup 106
57. Slow Cooker Taco Soup 108

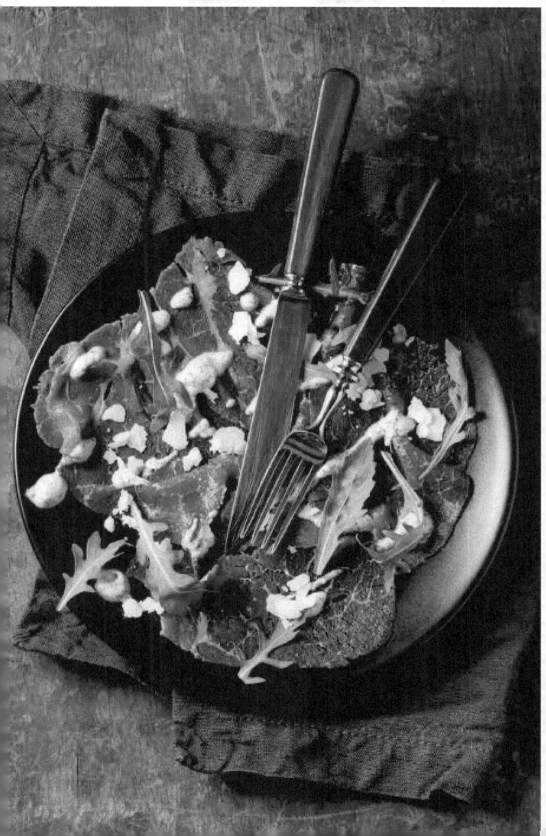

1. Parmesan Beef Slices

Preparation Time: 15 minutes

Cooking Time: 25 minutes

Servings: 4

Ingredients:

- 12 oz. beef brisket

- 1 teaspoon kosher salt

- 7 oz. Parmesan, sliced

- 5 oz. chive stems

- 1 teaspoon of turmeric

- 1 teaspoon of dried oregano

- 2 teaspoons of butter

Directions:

1. Preheat the air fryer to 365° F.

2. Meanwhile, slice the beef brisket into four slices, and sprinkle every beef slice with the turmeric and dried oregano.

3. Grease the air fryer's basket tray with the butter and put the beef slices inside.

4. Dice the chives and make a layer of it over the beef slices.

5. Make another layer using the Parmesan cheese, and cook the beef slices for 25 minutes.

6. Serve and enjoy!

Nutrition: Calories 348, Fat 18, Carbs 5, Protein 42,1.

2.   Sloppy Ground Beef Joes

Preparation Time: 5 minutes

Cooking Time: 25 minutes

Servings: 4

Ingredients:
- 1 ½ pound of lean ground beef
- ½ cup of green bell pepper (diced)
- 2 tablespoons of tomato paste
- 1 teaspoon of powdered stevia
- 1 tablespoon of yellow mustard
- 1 tablespoon of garlic and spring onion seasoning or salt, pepper, crushed garlic, garlic powder, and onion to taste
- ½ tablespoon of cinnamon chipotle seasoning (or use chipotle paste, ground cinnamon, and garlic)
- 1 tablespoon of red wine vinegar
- 1 cup of beef broth (low sodium)
- Salt and pepper

Directions:
1. In a skillet, add the beef and cook over medium heat for about 7 min.

2. While cooking, break the beef into smaller pieces and then add all ingredients except the broth and stir thoroughly to combine well.

3. Finally, add the broth and increase the heat to medium-high heat.

4. When it boils, lower the heat to low and simmer for about 15 minutes with the pot uncovered.

5. Serve hot into bowls and enjoy!

Nutrition: Calories 302, Fat 11,5, Fiber 0,6, Carbs 2,7, Protein 44,1.

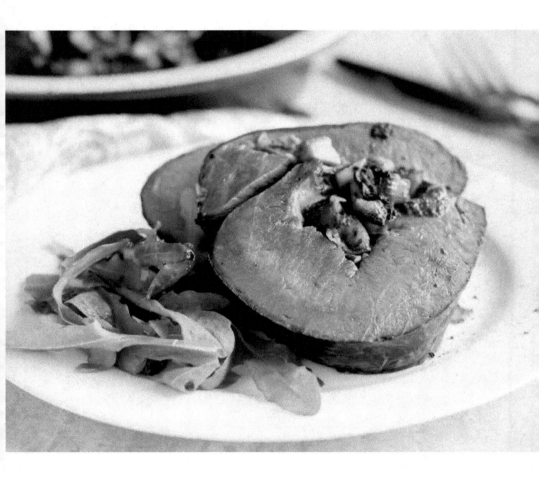

3. Spinach Beef Heart

Preparation Time: 15 minutes

Cooking Time: 20 minutes

Servings: 4

Ingredients:

- 1-pound beef heart

- 5 oz. chive stems

- ½ cup fresh spinach

- 1 teaspoon salt

- 1 teaspoon ground black pepper

- 3 cups chicken stock

- 1 teaspoon butter

Directions:

1. Preheat the air fryer to 400 °F.

2. Dice the chives and chop the fresh spinach.

3. Combine the chives diced, chopped spinach, and butter and stir.

4. Remove all the fat from the beef heart, make an incision on it, and fill it with the spinach-chives mixture.

5. Pour the chicken stock into the air fryer's basket tray.

6. Season the stuffed beef heart with the salt and ground black pepper, put it in the air fryer, and cook for 20 minutes.

7. When it's cooked, remove the heart from the air fryer, slice it and serve with the remaining liquid from the air fryer.

Nutrition: Calories 216, Fat 6,8, Fiber 0,8, Carbs 3,8, Protein 33,3.

4.   Taco Tasty Bowls

Preparation Time: 5 minutes

Cooking Time: 20 minutes

Servings: 4

Ingredients:
- 1 large head of cauliflower (ready-to-cook cauliflower rice)
- 1 ½ pound of lean ground beef
- 1-2 capfuls southwestern seasoning (or use low-salt taco seasoning)
- 2 cups of no-sugar, no-flavor added tomatoes (canned, diced)
- Favorite condiments

Directions:
1. In a skillet, add the ground beef and saute for about 12 min over medium-high heat, or until it turns slightly brown, breaking it into smaller pieces.

2. Add the seasoning, tomatoes, and stir thoroughly, then lower the heat to low and cook for an extra 5 min, or until the liquid reduces by half.

3. Meanwhile, chop the cauliflower to make cauliflower rice.

4. Season the beef mixture and the cauliflower rice and finally serve!

Nutrition: Calories 275, Fat 9,9, Fiber 2,3, Carbs 6,2, Protein 39.

5.   Quick and Easy Mongolian Beef

Preparation Time: 5 minutes

Cooking Time: 20 minutes

Servings: 8-10
Ingredients:
*   1 lb flank steak thinly sliced against the grain
*   2 Tbsp cornstarch
*   2-4 Tbsp canola oil
*   1 yellow onion sliced
*   2 green onions chopped, green and white parts separated
*   4 garlic cloves chopped
*   inch ginger chopped
*   ¼ c. low sodium soy sauce
*   ¼ c. water
*   1 Tbsp hoisin sauce
*   3 Tbsp brown sugar
*   Salt to taste

Directions:
1. Cover the flank steak with cornstarch and then set aside.

2. In a large skillet, heat the canola oil over medium-high heat, and then add the flank steak to the frying pan in a single layer, making sure that the pieces are not touching.

3. Cook for 1-2 minutes per side until each side is browned and all the flank steak is cooked and then set aside.

4. Into the skillet, add the sliced yellow onion, whites of green onions, garlic, and ginger and fry for about 3 minutes, until the onions are slightly softened but still have a little crunch.

5. Add soy sauce, water, hoisin sauce, and brown sugar and stir.

6. Finally reintroduce steak back to the skillet along with the green parts of the onions, remove from heat and serve. Enjoy!

Nutrition: Calories 303, Fat 13, Fiber 1, Carbs 20, Protein 26.

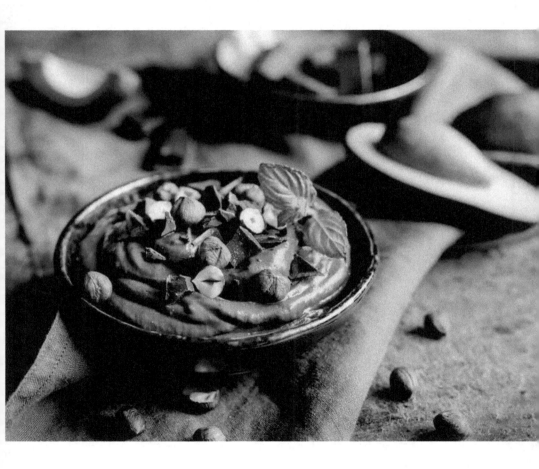

6.   Rich Chocolate Mousse

Preparation Time: 10 minutes

Cooking Time: 15 minutes

Servings: 3

Ingredients:

- ¼ cup of low-fat coconut cream

- 2 cups of fat-free Greek-style yogurt, strained

- 4 tsp. powered cocoa, no added sugar

- 2 tbsp. stevia/xylitol/bacon syrup

- 1 tsp. natural vanilla extract

Directions:

1. Into a bowl, combine all the ingredients and mix well.

2. Distribute the mixture into single-serving cups and let it rest in the refrigerator.

3. Once they're cold, serve and enjoy.

Nutrition: Calories 269, Fat 3, Carbs 20, Protein 43.

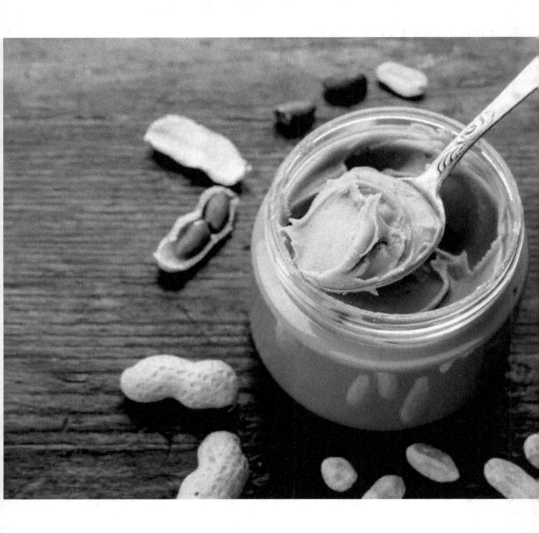

7.   Smooth Peanut Butter Cream

Preparation Time: 10 minutes

Cooking Time: 0

Servings: 8

Ingredients:

- ¼ cup of peanut butter

- 4 overripe bananas, chopped

- 1/3 cup cocoa powder

- ¼ tsp. vanilla extract

- 1/8 tsp. salt

Directions:

1. Into a blender, add all the ingredients, and blend until it's smooth.

2. Serve the smoothie immediately and enjoy or leave to cool in the fridge for 15 minutes and enjoy cold.

Nutrition: Calories 101, Fat 5, Carbs 14, Protein 3.

8.   Vanilla Avocado Popsicles

Preparation Time: 20 minutes

Cooking Time: 0

Servings: 6

Ingredients:

- 2 avocados

- 1 tsp. vanilla

- 1 cup of almond milk

- 1 tsp. liquid stevia

- ½ cup of unsweetened cocoa powder

Directions:

1. Into a blender, add all the ingredients, and blend until it's smooth.

2. Pour the mixture into the popsicle molds and place in the freezer until set.

3. Once they're cold, serve and enjoy.

Nutrition: Calories 130, Fat 12, Carbs 7, Protein 3.

9. Vanilla Bean Frappuccino

Preparation Time: 3 minutes

Cooking Time: 6 minutes

Servings: 4

Ingredients:

- 3 cups unsweetened vanilla almond milk, chilled

- 2 tsp. swerve

- 1 ½ cups heavy cream, cold

- 1 vanilla bean

- ¼ tsp. xanthan gum

- Unsweetened chocolate shavings to garnish

Directions:

1. In a blender, combine the almond milk, swerve, heavy cream, vanilla bean, and xanthan gum and blend on high speed for 1 minute until it's smooth.

2. Pour the mixture into tall glasses and sprinkle with chocolate shavings on the top. Enjoy!

Nutrition: Calories 193, Fat 14, Carbs 6, Protein 15.

10. Vegan Pumpkin Pie Chia Pudding

Preparation Time: 10 minutes

Cooking Time: 1 hour

Servings: 6

Ingredients:

- 3 cups unsweetened cashew milk

- 1 ½ cup canned pumpkin

- 1 tsp cinnamon

- ½ tsp ginger

- ½ tsp nutmeg

- 2 tsp vanilla extract

- ¼ tsp cloves

- 6 tbsp of chia seeds

- 3 tbsp maple syrup or sweetener of choice

Directions:

1. Into a blender, combine milk, pumpkin and all spices and mix well until it's smooth.

2. Add in the smoothie the chia seeds, stir, and refrigerate overnight.

3. The next morning re-stir, divide into portions and serve.

11.   Yogurt Mint

Preparation Time: 5 minutes

Cooking Time: 20 minutes

Servings: 8-10

Ingredients:

- 1 cup of onion slices
- ¼ cup of Chicken broth (low sodium)
- 4 tablespoon of balsamic vincotto (or use a balsamic reduction - do not use vinegar)
- Pinch of sea salt and fresh peppercorns

Directions:

1. In a pan, add the broth and onions and cook over medium heat for about 20 minutes without browning.

2. When the onions have become soft, add the balsamic vinegar.

3. Turn off the stove and stir gently; let the onions soak in the balsamic and then serve.

Note: Can be stored in the refrigerator for up to 1 week.

Nutrition: Calories 6, Fat 0, Fiber 0,2, Carbs 1,4, Protein 0,1.

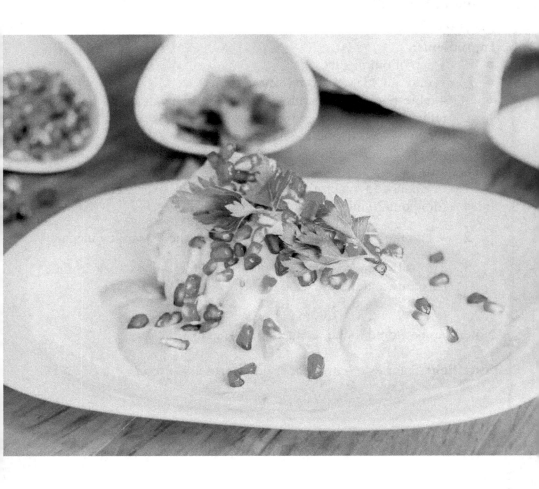

12. Cod Poblano Cream Sauce

Preparation Time: 15 minutes

Cooking Time: 20 minutes

Servings: 4

Ingredients:

- 2 green -5.5 ounces of Poblano peppers seeded and sliced
- 1 cup of sour cream
- 1 tablespoon of garlic and spring onion seasoning (or use fresh garlic, sea salt, parsley, and scallions)
- 5 cups of riced cauliflower (uncooked)
- ¼ cup of water
- 2 pounds of flaky white fish (use flounder, cod)

Directions:

1. Preheat the oven to 375 degrees.

2. Place the dressing, sour cream, and pepper in the food processor and blend to mix well.

3. Add the cauliflower to a baking dish, cover it in a single layer with the fish, and season with a pinch of pepper and salt.

4. Spread the mixture evenly over the fish and gently add the water to the cauliflower.

5. Bake for about 35 minutes until the fish is well cooked.

6. Remove from the oven, divide into 4 portions, and serve.

Nutrition: Calories 122, Fat 14, Carbs 2, Protein 23.

13. Coleslaw worth a Second Helping

Preparation Time: 20 minutes

Cooking Time: 0 minutes

Servings: 6
Ingredients:

- 5 cups shredded cabbage

- 2 carrots, shredded

- ½ cup mayonnaise

- ½ cup sour cream

- 3 tablespoons apple cider vinegar

- 1 teaspoon kosher salt

- ½ teaspoon celery seed

Directions:

1. In a large bowl, combine the cabbage, carrots, and parsley.

2. In another bowl, whisk together the mayonnaise, sour cream, vinegar, salt, and celery until smooth.

3. Pour the sauce over the vegetables until covered, transfer to a serving bowl and serve.

Nutrition: Calories 192, Fat 18, Fiber 3, Carbs 7, Protein 2.

14.   Fennel and Arugula Salad with Fig Vinaigrette

Preparation Time: 15 minutes

Cooking Time: 10 minutes

Servings: 6
Ingredients:

- 5 ounces of washed and dried arugula

- 1 small fennel bulb, it can be either shaved or tiny sliced

- 2 tablespoons of extra virgin oil or any cooking oil

- 1 teaspoon of lemon zest

- ½ teaspoon of salt

- Pepper (freshly ground)

- Pecorino

Directions:
1. In a serving bowl, mix the rocket and flaked fennel.

2. In another bowl, mix the olive or cooking oil, lemon zest, salt, and pepper, shake until creamy and smooth.

3. Pour and season over the salad, stirring gently to blend.

4. Cut a few slices of pecorino, lay it on top of the salad, and serve.

Nutrition: Calories 85,7 - Fat 9,7, Fiber 3,4, Carbs 14,3, Protein 2,1.

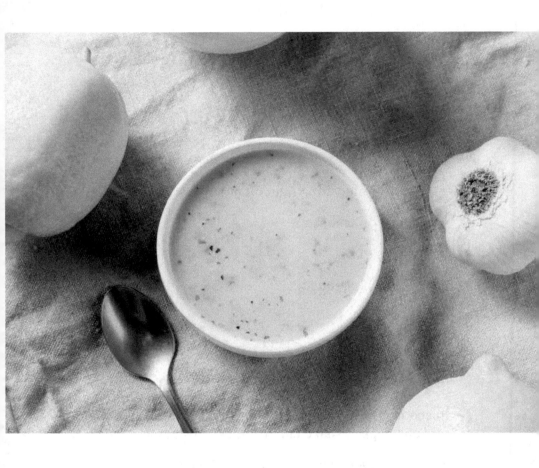

15. Garlic Vinaigrette

Preparation Time: 10 minutes

Cooking Time: 30 minutes

Servings: 1

Ingredients:
- 1 clove garlic, crushed
- 4 tablespoons olive oil
- 1 tablespoon lemon juice
- Freshly ground black pepper

Directions:
1. Simply mix all the ingredients. Serve or refrigerate.

Nutrition: Calories 104, Fat 3,1, Fiber 1,3, Carbs 16,2, Protein 1,3.

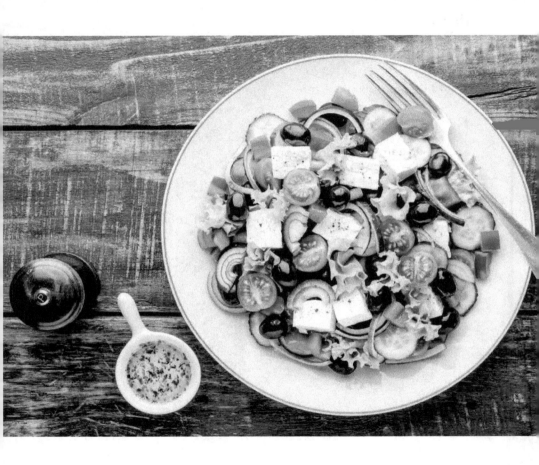

16. Greek Salad

Preparation Time: 15 minutes

Cooking Time: 15 minutes

Servings: 5

Ingredients:

FOR DRESSING:

- ½ teaspoon black pepper

- ¼ teaspoon salt

- ½ teaspoon oregano

- 1 tablespoon garlic powder

- 2 tablespoons balsamic vinegar

- 1/3 cup olive oil

FOR SALAD:

- ½ cup sliced black olives

- ½ cup chopped parsley, fresh

- 1 small red onion, thin-sliced

- 1 cup cherry tomatoes, sliced

- 1 bell pepper, yellow, chunked

- 1 cucumber, peeled, quarter and slice

- 4 cups chopped romaine lettuce

- ½ teaspoon salt

- 2 tablespoons olive oil

Directions:
1. In a small container, mix all the ingredients for the dressing and let it rest in the refrigerator.

2. In a large bowl and mix the vegetables, pour the dressing over the salad, and serve.

Nutrition: Calories 234, Fat 16,1, Carbs 48, Protein 5.

17. Green Beans

Preparation Time: 5 minutes

Cooking Time: 13 minutes

Servings: 4

Ingredients:

- 1-pound green beans

- ¾ teaspoon garlic powder

- ¾ teaspoon ground black pepper

- 1 ¼ teaspoon salt

- ½ teaspoon paprika

Directions:

1. Preheat the deep fryer at 400 °F for 5 minutes.

2. Meanwhile, place the beans into a bowl, sprinkle with olive oil, garlic powder, black pepper, salt, and paprika and mix until well coated.

3. Open the air fryer, add the green beans, close with the lid and cook for 8 minutes until golden and crisp, stirring halfway through cooking.

4. When cooked, transfer the green beans to a serving dish and serve.

Nutrition: Calories 45, Fat 11, Fiber 3, Carbs 2, Protein 4.

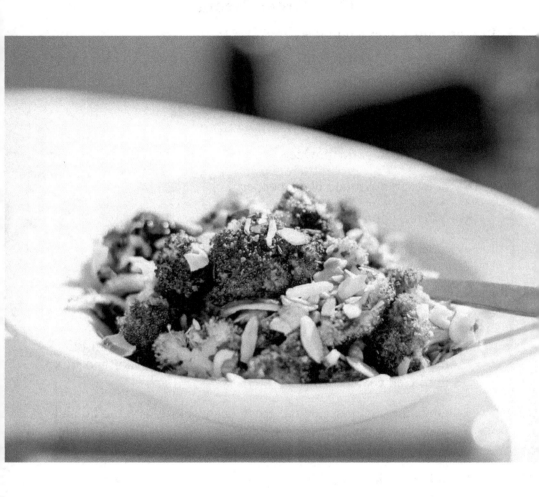

18. Healthy Broccoli Salad

Preparation Time: 5 minutes

Cooking Time: 25 minutes

Servings: 6

Ingredients:

- 3 cups broccoli, chopped

- 1 tbsp. apple cider vinegar

- ½ cup Greek yogurt

- 2 tbsp. sunflower seeds

- 3 bacon slices, cooked and chopped

- 1/3 cup onion, sliced

- 1/4 tsp. stevia

Directions:

1. In a mixing bowl, mix the broccoli, onion, and bacon.

2. In a small bowl, mix the yogurt, vinegar, and stevia and pour over the broccoli mixture.

3. Mix well and sprinkle the sunflower seeds over the salad.

4. Keep the salad in the refrigerator for 30 minutes, then serve and enjoy.

Nutrition: Calories 90, Fat 4,9, Carbs 5,4, Protein 6,2.

19. Kohlrabi Cilantro slaw

Preparation Time: 25 minutes

Cooking Time: 0 minutes

Servings: 8
Ingredients:
- 4 cups of Kohlrabi (sliced into matchsticks)
- ¼ cup of cilantro (chopped)
- 1 teaspoon of no-salt taco seasoning
- 1 teaspoon of cajun seasoning (garlic use a mixture of any of garlic, cumin, salt, onion, cayenne pepper, and black pepper)
- 1 lime (zest)
- 1 orange (zest)
- 1 lime juice
- 4 teaspoons of orange oil (or your favorite oil and fresh-squeezed orange juice)

Directions:
1. Into a bowl, add all ingredients (except cilantro and kohlrabi) and whisk together.

2. Add the kohlrabi and sprinkle with coriander.

3. Mix with two spoons and leave to rest in the fridge for at least 15 minutes before serving.

Nutrition: Calories 38, Fat 2,3, Fiber 2,5, Carbs 4,2, Protein 1,2.

20. Lemon Caper Pesto

Preparation Time: 10 minutes

Cooking Time: 10 minutes

Servings: 1
Ingredients:

- 6 tablespoons of fresh parsley leaves

- 3 cloves of garlic

- 2 tablespoons of capers

- 2 oz. cashew nuts

- 2 tablespoons of olive oil

- 1 tablespoon of lemon juice

Directions:

1. Place all of the ingredients into a food processor and blitz until smooth and if necessary, add a little extra oil.

2. Serve with pasta, vegetables, or meat dishes.

Nutrition: Calories 250, Fat 4,1, Fiber 1,6, Carbs 16,4, Protein 1,5.

21. Lemon Kale Cider Vinegar

Preparation Time: 5 minutes

Cooking Time: 20 minutes

Servings: 8-10

Ingredients:

- 1 pound of fresh kale (wash & remove ribs)

- 4 teaspoons of lemon oil (you can use orange or roasted garlic oil)

- ¼ cup of apple cider vinegar

- ½ tablespoon of Thai seasoning(or use a mixture of garlic, lemongrass, onion, red pepper, Thai basil, lime, and salt)

- ¼ c of Dry cranberries (you can use apples or orange segments)

Directions:

1. In a food processor, add the kale and whisk until well chopped.

2. Add other ingredients and blend well.

3. Leave to rest in the fridge before serving.

Nutrition: Calories 22, Fat 0,6, Fiber 0,6, Carbs 3,7, Protein 1.

22.   Lime Cilantro crema

Preparation Time: 10 minutes

Cooking Time: 0 minutes

Servings: 4
Ingredients:
- 1 cup of Sour cream
- Seasoning (a mixture of garlic, salt, onion, and pepper) - to taste
- 1 lime zest
- 1 lime juice
- ¼ cup of fresh cilantro (finely shredded)

Directions:
1. Add all the ingredients to a bowl and stir thoroughly to combine well.

2. Allow to settle for about 15 minutes, then serve.

Note: It can be stored in the refrigerator for up to a week with an airtight container.

Nutrition: Calories 27, Fat 2,5, Fiber 0,1, Carbs 1, Protein 0,4.

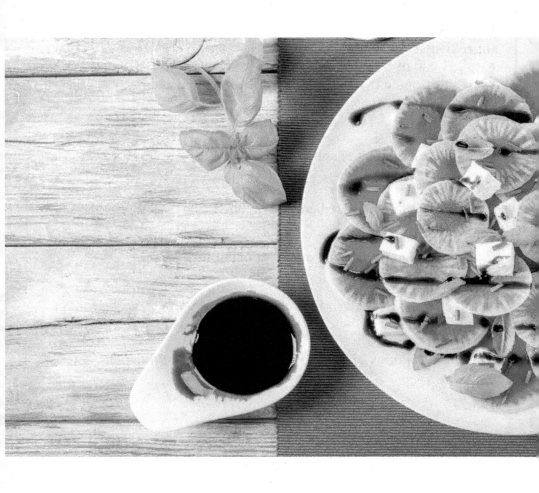

23. Mozzarella Radish Salad

Preparation Time: 10 minutes

Cooking Time: 20 minutes

Servings: 2

Ingredients:

- 8 oz. radish

- 4 oz. Mozzarella

- 1 teaspoon of balsamic vinegar

- ½ teaspoon salt

- 1 tablespoon olive oil

- 1 teaspoon dried oregano

Directions:

1. Wash the radish carefully and cut it into halves.

2. Preheat the air fryer to 360 °F.

3. Put the radish halves in the air fryer basket, sprinkle the radish with salt and olive oil, and cook it for 20 minutes.

4. Shake the radish after 10 minutes of cooking.

5. When the time is over, transfer the radish to the serving plate, chop Mozzarella roughly and sprinkle the radish with Mozzarella, balsamic vinegar, and dried oregano.

6. Stir it gently and serve it immediately.

Nutrition: Calories 241, Fat 17,2, Fiber 2,1, Carbs 6,4, Protein 16,9.

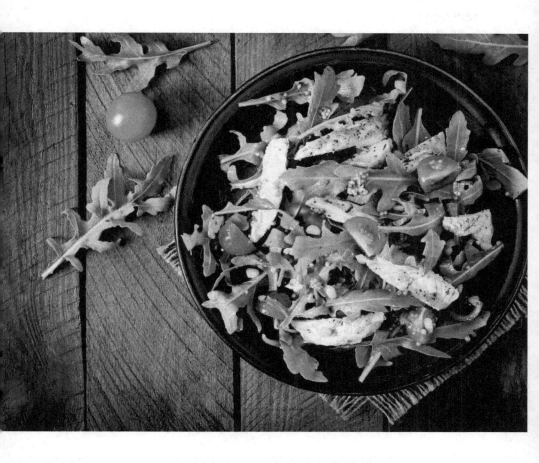

24. Mediterranean Chicken Salad

Preparation Time: 15 minutes

Cooking Time: 30 minutes

Servings: 4

Ingredients:

FOR CHICKEN:

- 1 3/4 lb. boneless, skinless chicken breast

- ¼ teaspoon each of pepper and salt (or as desired)

- 1 ½ tablespoon of butter, melted

FOR MEDITERRANEAN SALAD:

- 1 cup of sliced cucumber

- 6 cups of romaine lettuce, that is torn or roughly chopped 10 pitted Kalamata olives

- 10 pint of cherry tomatoes

- 1/3 cup of reduced-fat feta cheese

- ¼ teaspoon each of pepper and salt (or lesser)

- 1 small lemon juice (it should be about 2 tablespoons)

Directions:

1. Preheat your oven or grill to about 350°F.

2. Season the chicken with salt, butter, and black pepper and roast or grill chicken until it reaches an internal temperature of 165°F in about 25 minutes.

3. Once your chicken breasts are cooked, remove and keep aside to rest for about 5 minutes before you slice them.

4. Meanwhile, combine all the salad ingredients you have, toss everything together very well, and serve the chicken with the Mediterranean salad.

Nutrition: Calories 340, Fat 14, Carbs 9, Protein 45.

25. Mini Zucchini Bites

Preparation Time: 10 minutes

Cooking Time: 10 minutes

Servings: 6
Ingredients:

- 1 zucchini, cut into thick circles

- 3 cherry tomatoes, halved

- ½ cup of Parmesan cheese,

- grated Salt and pepper to taste

- 1 tsp. chives, chopped

Directions:

1. Preheat the oven to 390 °F and add greaseproof paper to a baking sheet.

2. Arrange the courgette pieces on the baking sheet and add the cherry halves to each courgette slice.

3. Add the parmesan, chives, sprinkle with salt and pepper, and cook for 10 minutes. Serve and enjoy!

Nutrition: Calories 52,8 - Fat 1, Carbs 7,3.

26. Nicoise Salad

Preparation Time: 15 minutes

Cooking Time: 10 minutes

Servings: 4

Ingredients:
- 1 oz. red potatoes
- 1 package of green beans
- 2 eggs
- ½ cup tomatoes
- 2 tablespoons wine vinegar
- ¼ teaspoon salt
- ½ teaspoon pepper
- ½ teaspoon thyme
- ¼ cup olive oil
- 6 oz. of tuna
- ¼ cup Kalamata olives

Directions:
1. Into a bowl, combine all ingredients, add salad dressing, and serve.

Nutrition: Calories 189, Fat 7, Fiber 2, Carbs 2, Protein 15.

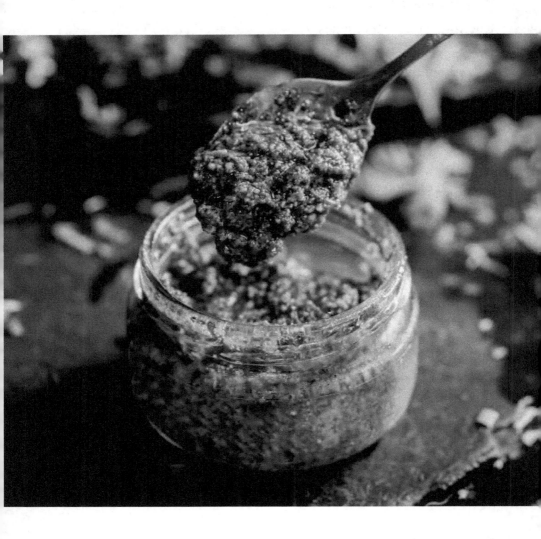

27. Parsley Pesto

Preparation Time: 10 minutes

Cooking Time: 10 minutes

Servings: 1

Ingredients:

- 3 oz. Parmesan cheese, finely grated

- 2 oz. pine nuts

- 6 tablespoons fresh parsley leaves, chopped

- 2 cloves of garlic

- 2 tablespoons olive oil

Directions:

1. Put all the ingredients in a food processor and blend until you get a smooth and homogeneous paste.

Nutrition: Calories 104, Fat 4,3, Fiber 1,6, Carbs 16,2, Protein 1,3.

28.   Pico de Gallo Salad

Preparation Time: 15 minutes

Cooking Time: 0 minutes

Servings: 2
Ingredients:
- 1 cup of diced tomatoes
- ¼ cup of onion (chopped)
- 1 teaspoon of seasoning (or a mixture of garlic, salt, onion, pepper to taste)
- 2 tablespoons of cilantro (finely chopped)
- 1 lime juice

Directions:
1. Into a bowl, add all the ingredients, mix well, and leave to rest for about 15 minutes in the refrigerator.

Note: You can refrigerate up to a week with an airtight container.

Nutrition: Calories 20, Fat 0,2, Fiber 1,2, Carbs 16,2, Protein 1,3.

29. Portobello Italiano Sausage

Preparation Time: 5 minutes

Cooking Time: 20 minutes

Servings: 4
Ingredients:

- 4 Portobello mushrooms (large)

- 1 ½ pound 86-95% lean Italian sausage

- 1 tablespoon of garlic & spring onion seasoning (or use chopped chives, chopped garlic, onion powder, garlic powder, salt, and pepper)

Directions:

1. Preheat the oven to 350 degrees.

2. Wash the stems and caps of the mushrooms and cut the stems of them.

3. Add the other ingredients to a bowl and mix well.

4. With the smooth side facing down, place the mushroom caps on a baking sheet.

5. Divide the mixture equally into 4 portions and arrange it on the mushroom caps.

6. Place in the oven and cook for about 25 minutes, then serve.

Nutrition: Calories 244, Fat 12,7, Fiber 0, Carbs 8, Protein 23,1.

30. Quinoa with Vegetables

Preparation Time: 10 minutes

Cooking Time: 5 hours

Servings: 8

Ingredients:

- 2 cups quinoa, rinsed and drained

- 2 onions, chopped

- 2 carrots, peeled and sliced

- 1 cup of sliced cremini mushrooms

- 3 garlic cloves, minced

- 4 cups low-sodium vegetable broth

- ½ teaspoon of salt

- 1 teaspoon of dried marjoram leaves

- 1/8 teaspoon of freshly ground black pepper

Directions:

1. In a 6-quart slow cooker, mix all of the ingredients, cover, and cook on low for 5 to 6 hours, or until the quinoa and vegetables are tender.

2. Stir the mixture and serve.

Nutrition: Calories 204, Fat 3, Fiber 4, Carbs 35, Protein 7.

31. Romaine Lettuce and Radicchios Mix

Preparation Time: 6 minutes

Cooking Time: 0 minutes

Servings: 4

Ingredients:

- 2 tablespoons of olive oil

- A pinch of salt and black pepper

- 2 spring onions, chopped

- 3 tablespoons Dijon mustard

- Juice of 1 lime

- ½ cup basil, chopped

- 4 cups romaine lettuce heads, chopped

- 3 radicchios, sliced

Directions:

1. In a salad bowl, blend all ingredients, serve and enjoy!

Nutrition: Calories 87, Fat 2, Fiber 1, Carbs 1, Protein 2.

32. Rosemary Creamy Fauxtatoes

Preparation Time: 5 minutes

Cooking Time: 30 minutes

Servings: 4

Ingredients:

- 1 ½ lb of sirloin steak (cubed into 1-inch chunks)
- 1 tablespoon of rosemary seasoning (or use a mixture of fresh rosemary, garlic, sage, onion, and black pepper)
- 2 ½ cups of beef broth (low sodium)
- 4 cups of baby portobello mushrooms (sliced)
- 1 tablespoon of garlic and spring onion seasoning (or use a mixture of scallions, minced garlic, pepper, and salt
- 1 teaspoon of Seasoning (or use pepper and salt)
- ½ tsp of guar gum (or other approved thickener)
- ¼ cup of water
- 2 cups of cauliflower mashed potatoes (hot)

Directions:

1. Add all ingredients (except cauliflower mashed potatoes and guar gum) to a pressure cooker, mix well and cook over high heat for about 15 minutes.

2. When finished, quickly release the pressure, remove the lid, and brown.

3. Mix the guar gum and water thoroughly without lumps and, when the mixture in the pot starts to boil, add the gum mixture and mix.

4. Cook for about 5 minutes or until the sauce becomes thick. Season with salt and serve.

Nutrition: Calories 341, Fat 11,6, Fiber 1,3, Carbs 4,1, Protein 51,5.

33. Shrimp Cobb Salad

Preparation Time: 25 minutes

Cooking Time: 10 minutes

Servings: 2

Ingredients:

- 4 slices center-cut bacon

- 1 lb. large shrimp, peeled and deveined

- ½ teaspoon of ground paprika

- ¼ teaspoon of ground black pepper

- ¼ teaspoon of salt, divided

- 2 ½ tablespoons fresh lemon juice

- 1 ½ tablespoon of extra-virgin olive oil

- ½ teaspoon of whole-grain Dijon mustard

- (10 oz.) package romaine lettuce hearts, chopped

- 2 cups cherry tomatoes, quartered

- 1 ripe avocado, cut into wedges

- 1 cup shredded carrots

Directions:

1. In a skillet, cook the bacon for 4 minutes until crisp, then place it on absorbent paper and allow to cool for 5 minutes.

2. Remove the fat from the bacon, leaving only 1 tablespoon in the pan.

3. Heat the skillet over medium-high heat and in the meantime, season the shrimp with black pepper and paprika.

4. Cook the shrimp for about 2 minutes per side until opaque, then sprinkle with 1/8 teaspoon of salt for seasoning.

5. Combine the remaining 1/8 teaspoon of salt, mustard, olive oil, and lemon juice in a small bowl and mix.

6. On each serving dish, arrange 1 ½ cups of romaine lettuce. Add the same amounts of avocado, carrots, tomatoes, shrimp, and bacon on top. Serve and enjoy!

Nutrition: Calories 528, Fat 28,7, Carbs 22,7, Protein 48,9.

34.   Stewed Herbed Fruit

Preparation Time: 15 minutes

Cooking Time: 6 hours

Servings: 12
Ingredients:

- 2 cups dried apricots

- 2 cups prunes

- 2 cups dried pears

- 2 cups dried apples

- 1 cup dried cranberries

- ¼ cup honey

- 6 cups of water

- 1 teaspoon dried thyme leaves

- 1 teaspoon dried basil leaves

Directions:
1. In a 6-quart slow cooker, mix all ingredients, cover, and cook over low heat for 6-8 hours, or until fruits have absorbed liquid and are tender.

Notes: Can be stored in the refrigerator for up to 1 week.

Nutrition: Calories 242, Fat 0, Fiber 9, Carbs 61, Protein 2.

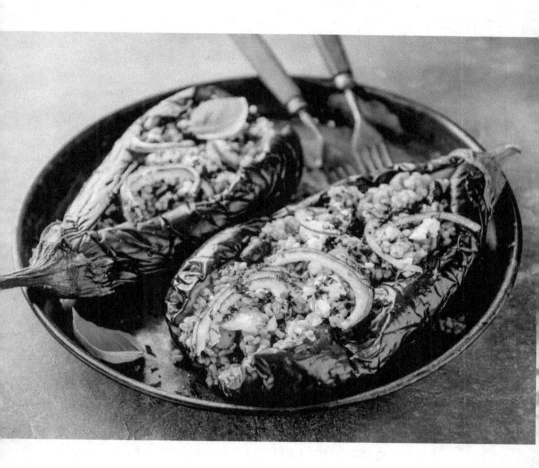

35. Stuffed Eggplant Provencale

Preparation Time: 15 minutes

Cooking Time: 40 minutes

Servings: 4
Ingredients:
- 2 small eggplants (you can use zucchini)
- Sea salt –to taste
- 4 tsp of roasted garlic oil (or use any oil of choice and fresh garlic)
- 2 lbs of lean ground garlic
- 1 tablespoon of garlic and spring onion seasoning (or a mixture of garlic, parsley, onion, paprika, and lemon)
- 1 cup of fresh tomatoes (diced and well-drained)
- ½ cup of zucchini (chopped into ½" Cubes)
- ½ cup of mushrooms (sliced)
- 1 cup of chicken stock (low sodium)

Directions:
1. Preheat the oven to 350.

2. In lengthwise, cut the eggplants into halves. Scoop out the seed with a spoon and discard.

3. Remove the zucchini flesh with your spoon and make a shell with ¾ inch thick sides. Dice the removed flesh, set it aside, and sprinkle over the shell with a little salt and set it aside.

4. Heat the garlic oil until it sizzles, then add the turkey with the diced eggplant to the pan and cook for about 5 min, or until the turkey turns opaque. Stir occasionally.

5. Add the garlic seasoning and veggies and cook for an extra 1minute.

6. Rinse the salted eggplant halves and pat dry, then with the hollow side facing up, place the halves on baking dishes.

7. Scoop equal portions of the turkey mixture into eggplant shells, pour the remaining stock into the baking dish, and place them in the oven (middle rack).

8. Bake for about 40 min, or until the eggplant becomes tender. Serve and enjoy!

Nutrition: Calories 320, Fat 5,3, Fiber 3,7, Carbs 7,3, Protein 62,4.

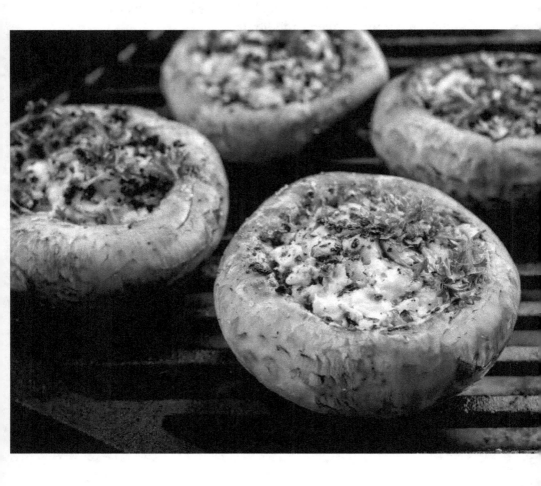

36.   Stuffed Mushrooms Feta

Preparation Time: 10 minutes

Cooking Time: 30 minutes

Servings: 4

Ingredients:

- 1 ½ pound of lean ground beef (or can use turkey, chicken, or lamb)

- 1 tablespoon of Mediterranean seasoning (or use a mixture of black pepper, basil, onion, oregano, parsley, rosemary, and sage)

- ¼ teaspoon of Seasoning (or use fresh pepper and sea salt)

- ½ cup of crumbled feta cheese

- 4 cups of Portobello mushroom

Directions:

1. Add the Mediterranean seasoning, beef, and feta into a bowl and mix to combine and divide the mixture into 4 equal meatballs.

2. Add the mushrooms caps to the baking dish and season with proper and salt.

3. Press the mixture into the mushrooms caps, place in the oven, and bake for about 30 minutes, or until it is well cooked.

Nutrition: Calories 308, Fat 11,9, Fiber 0,4, Carbs 1,7, Protein 46,1.

37. Taste of Normandy Salad

Preparation Time: 25 minutes

Cooking Time: 5 minutes

Servings: 4-6

Ingredients:

- 2 tablespoons butter

- ¼ cup sugar or honey

- 1 cup walnut pieces

- ½ teaspoon kosher salt

- 3 tablespoons of extra-virgin olive oil

- 1½ tablespoons champagne vinegar

- 1½ tablespoons Dijon mustard

- ¼ teaspoon kosher salt

- 1 head red leaf lettuce, shredded into pieces

- 3 heads endive, ends trimmed and leaves separated

- 2 apples, cored and divided into thin wedges

- 1 (8-ounce) Camembert wheel, cut into thin wedges

Directions:

1. Dissolve the butter in a skillet over medium-high heat and stir in the sugar and cook until it dissolves.

2. Add the walnuts and cook for about 5 minutes, stirring, until toasty.

---

3. Season with salt and transfer to a plate to cool.

4. Meanwhile, in a large bowl, whip the oil, vinegar, mustard, and salt until combined.

5. Add the lettuce and endive to the bowl with the dressing, and toss well, then transfer to a serving platter.

6. Decoratively arrange the apple and Camembert wedges over the lettuce, scatter the walnuts on top and serve immediately.

Nutrition: Calories 699, Fat 52, Fiber 17, Carbs 44, Protein 23.

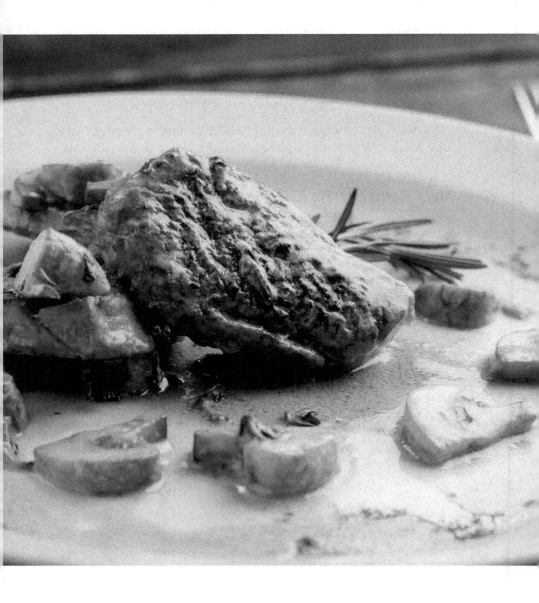

38. Tenderloins Mushrooms

Preparation Time: 10 minutes

Cooking Time: 25 minutes

Servings: 4

Ingredients:

- 1 teaspoon of Seasoning of choice (or a mixture of garlic, parsley, salt, black pepper, and onion)

- 1 ½ lb of pork tenderloin (you can use chicken breasts or beef tenderloin)

- 6 cups of Portobello mushroom caps (chopped into chunks)

- ½ chicken broth (low sodium)

- 1 tablespoon of garlic and spring onion seasoning (or a mixture of garlic, parsley, salt, onion, paprika, and black pepper)

- Fresh parsley (for garnish)

Directions:

1. Preheat the oven to 400 degrees and season both sides of the fillet.

2. Over high heat, place the baking sheet on the stove and grease it with non-stick cooking spray.

3. Once the pan has heated up, place the fillets in the pan without touching and cook each side for about 3 minutes or until brown.

4. Remove from the pan and set aside.

5. Leave the pan on the stove, add the broth, mushrooms, and garlic dressing.

6. Scrape the brown part off the bottom with the wooden spoon and cook the mixture for 1 more minute.

7. Return the pork to the pan and cook in the oven for about 25 min.

8. Remove from the oven and allow to cool for a few minutes, then slice the pork and serve with the sauce and mushrooms.

Nutrition: Calories 214, Fat 5, Fiber 0, Carbs 1,2, Protein 38,1.

39. Teriyaki Sauce

Preparation Time: 10 minutes

Cooking Time: 30 minutes

Servings: 1

Ingredients:

- 7 fl-oz soy sauce

- 7 fl-oz pineapple juice

- 1 teaspoon red wine vinegar

- 1-inch chunk of fresh ginger root, peeled and chopped

- 2 cloves of garlic

Directions:

1. Place the ingredients into a saucepan, bring them to a boil, then reduce the heat and simmer for 10 minutes.

2. Let it cool, then remove the garlic and ginger.

3. Store it in a container in the fridge until ready to use.

Note: Use as a marinade for meat, fish, and tofu dishes.

Nutrition: Calories 267, Fat 4,3, Fiber 1,2, Carbs 16,2, Protein 1,3.

40. Tomatoes Creamy Garlic Sauce

Preparation Time: 15 minutes

Cooking Time: 15 minutes

Servings: 4

Ingredients:
- 1 ½ pound of boneless sirloin steak (remove excess fat)
- 1 tablespoon of cajun seasoning (or any other blackening seasoning)
- 2 cups of fresh garden tomatoes (chopped)
- ½ cup of light sour cream
- 1 tablespoon of apple cider vinegar
- 1 tablespoon of garlic and spring onion seasoning (or use fresh garlic, parsley, onion, and lemon)
- Ground pepper and natural sea salt to taste

Directions:
1. Season the steak with the Cajun seasoning, then grill the steak on each side for about 7 minutes.

2. Meanwhile, make the sauce by mixing the sour cream, vinegar, and garlic dressing into a bowl.

3. Let the steak rest for about 5 minutes before slicing it.

4. Season the steak with 1 tablespoon of garlic sauce and serve with ½ cup of tomatoes as a side dish. Enjoy!

Nutrition: Calories 324, Fat 9,8, Fiber 1,1, Carbs 4, Protein 52,4.

41.   Turmeric & Lemon Dressing

Preparation Time: 10 minutes

Cooking Time: 30 minutes

Servings: 1
Ingredients:
- 1 teaspoon of turmeric

- 4 tablespoons of olive oil

- Juice of 1 lemon

Directions:
1. Combine all the ingredients into a bowl and serve with salads. Enjoy!

Nutrition: Calories 125, Fat 3,3, Fiber 1,6, Carbs 16,3, Protein 1,5.

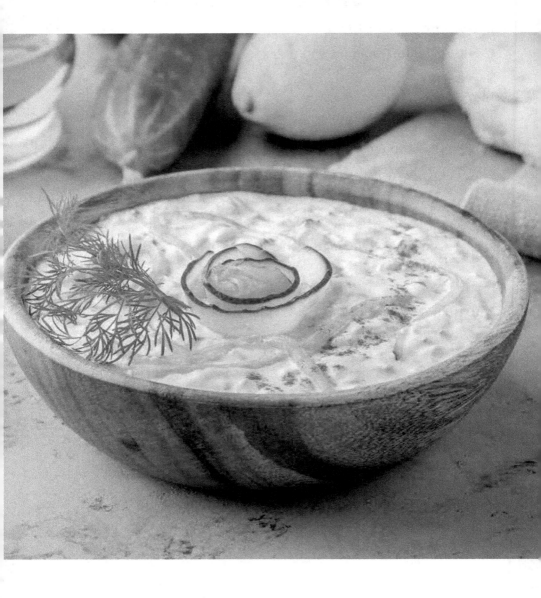

42. Tzatziki Salad

Preparation Time: 15 minutes

Cooking Time: 0 minutes

Servings: 4

Ingredients:

- 4 cups of fresh cucumbers (chopped)
- ½ cup of low-fat Greek yogurt
- ½ tablespoon of Seasoning (or use a mixture of garlic, lime, onion, parsley, lemon, and salt)
- 1 tablespoon of citrus dill seasoning (or garlic, onion, lemon, parsley, dill)

Directions:

1. Into a bowl, mix the spices and yogurt.

2. Add the cucumber and mix to coat well.

3. Leave the mixture to rest for about 15 minutes in the refrigerator, then serve and enjoy.

Nutrition: Calories 49, Fat 1, Fiber 0,6, Carbs 5,9, Protein 5,2.

43. Walnut & Mint Pesto

Preparation Time: 10 minutes

Cooking Time: 0 minutes

Servings: 1
Ingredients:
- 6 tablespoons fresh mint leaves
- 2oz walnuts
- 2 cloves of garlic
- 3½oz Parmesan cheese
- 1 tablespoon lemon juice

Directions:
1. Put all the ingredients into a food processor and blend until it becomes a smooth paste. Use as you wish!

Nutrition: Calories 99, Fat 4,4, Fiber 1,6, Carbs 16,4, Protein 1,6.

44. Walnut Vinaigrette

Preparation Time: 10 minutes

Cooking Time: 0 minutes

Servings: 1
Ingredients:

- 1 clove garlic, finely chopped

- 6 tablespoons of olive oil

- 3 tablespoons of red wine vinegar

- 1 tablespoon of walnut oil

- Sea salt

- Freshly ground black pepper

Directions:
1. Into a bowl, combine all of the ingredients and season with salt and pepper. Use immediately or store in the fridge.

Nutrition: Calories 109, Fat 4,3, Fiber 1,6, Carbs 16,4, Protein 1,6.

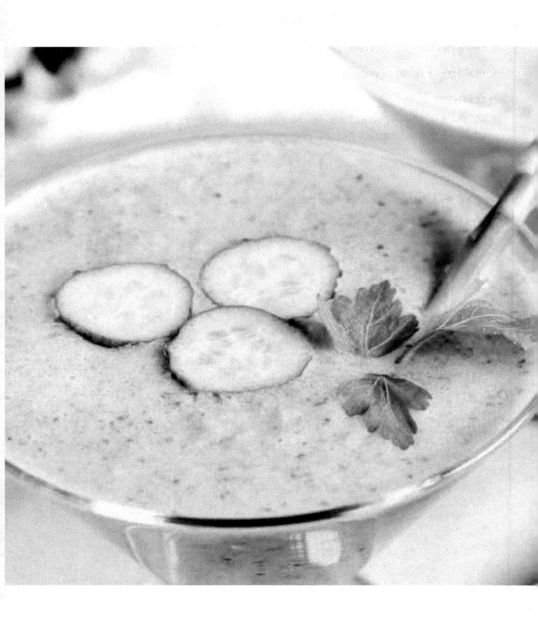

45. Asparagus Avocado Soup

Preparation time: 10 minutes

Cooking time: 20 minutes

Servings: 4

Ingredients:

- 1 avocado, peeled, pitted, cubed
- 12 ounces asparagus
- ½ teaspoon of ground black pepper
- 1 teaspoon of garlic powder
- 1 teaspoon of sea salt
- 2 tablespoons of olive oil, divided
- ½ of a lemon, juiced
- 2 cups of vegetable stock

Directions:

1. Preheat Air Fryer at 425 °F for 5 minutes.
2. Meanwhile, place asparagus in a shallow dish, drizzle with 1tablespoon oil, sprinkle with garlic powder, salt, and black pepper, and toss until well mixed.
3. In the air fryer, add the asparagus and cook them for 10 minutes until nicely golden and roasted, shaking after 5 minutes of cooking.
4. Once they're cooked, transfer asparagus into a food processor and combine the remaining ingredients. Pulse until well combined and smooth.

5. Tip the soup in a saucepan, (if the soup is too thick, add some water in) and heat it over medium-low heat for 5 minutes.

6. Ladle soup into bowls and serve hot.

Nutrition: Calories 208, Fat 11, Fiber 5, Carbs 2, Protein 4.

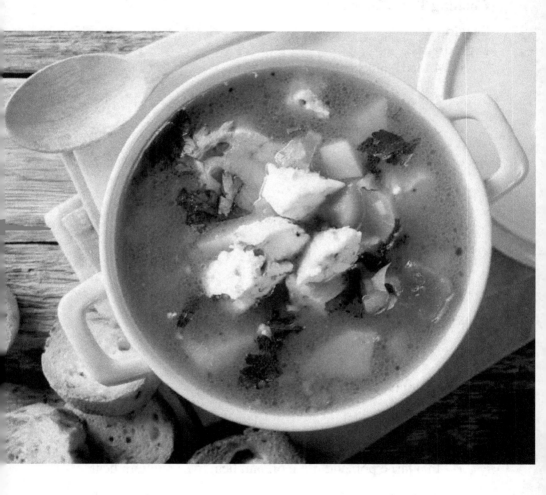

46. Buffalo Chicken Soup

Preparation Time: 20 minutes

Cooking Time: 20 minutes

Servings: 4

Ingredients:

- 4 med. stalks celery, diced

- 2 med. carrots, diced

- 4 chicken breasts, boneless & skinless

- 6 tbsp. butter

- 1 qt. chicken broth

- 2 oz. cream cheese

- ½ c. heavy cream

- ½ c. buffalo sauce

- 1 tsp. sea salt

- ½ tsp. thyme, dried

- Sour cream

- Green onions thinly sliced Bleu cheese crumbles

Directions:

1. In a large pot, add olive oil and heat over medium heat.

2. Add celery and carrot and cook them until shiny and tender. Then, add chicken breasts into the pot, cover, and allow cooking for about five to six minutes per side.

---

3. Once the chicken has cooked and formed some caramelization on each side, remove it from the pot. Shred the chicken breasts and set them aside.

4. Pour the chicken broth into the pot with the carrots and celery, then stir in the cream, butter, and cream cheese.

5. Bring the pot to a boil, and then add the chicken back to the pot.

6. Stir buffalo sauce into the mix and combine completely, then add seasonings, stir, and drop the heat to low and allow the soup to simmer for 15 to 20 minutes.

7. Serve hot with a garnish of sour cream, bleu cheese crumbles, and sliced green onion!

Nutrition: Calories 363, Fat 32,5, Carbs 4, Protein 57.

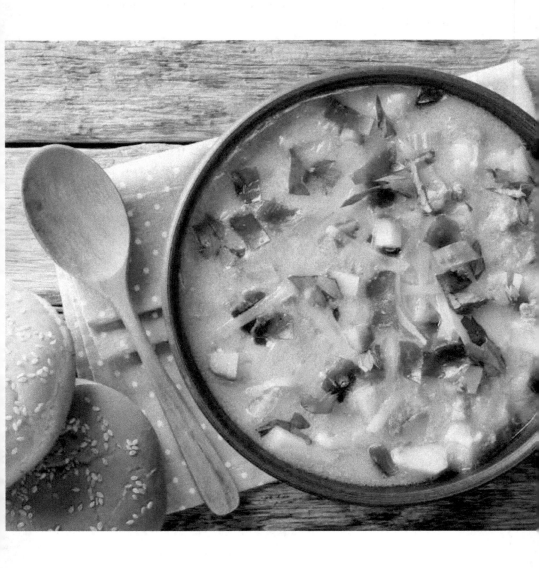

47. Cheeseburger Soup

Preparation Time: 15 minutes

Cooking Time: 45 minutes

Servings: 4

Ingredients:

- ¼ cup of chopped onion

- 1 quantity of 14.5 oz. can dice tomato

- 1 lb. of 90% lean ground beef

- 3/4 cup of chopped celery

- 2 teaspoons of Worcestershire sauce

- 3 cups of low sodium chicken broth

- ¼ teaspoon of salt

- 1 teaspoon of dried parsley

- 7 cups of baby spinach

- ¼ teaspoon of ground pepper

- 4 oz. of reduced-fat shredded cheddar cheese

Directions:
1. Brown the beef into a large soup pot and then add the celery, onion, and saute.

2. When they become soft, remove them from the heat and drain excess liquid.

85

3. Stir in the broth, tomatoes, parsley, Worcestershire sauce, pepper, and salt, cover with the lid and allow it to simmer on low heat for about 20 minutes.

4. Add spinach and leave it to cook until it becomes wilted for about 1-3 minutes.

5. Once the beef is cooked, top each of your servings with 1 ounce of cheese and serve.

Nutrition: Calories 400, Fat 20, Carbs 11, Protein 44.

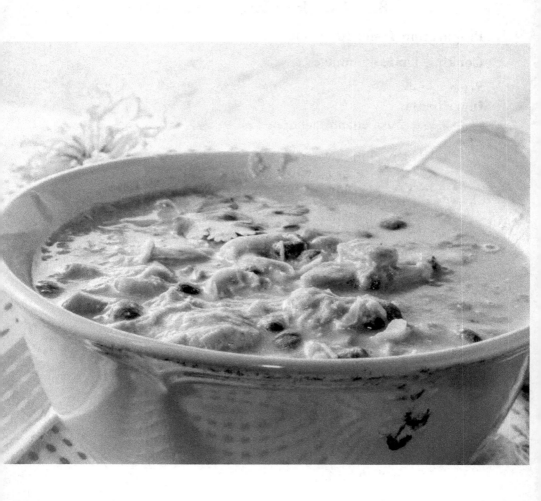

48.   Chicken Enchilada Soup

Preparation Time: 10 minutes

Cooking Time: 45 minutes

Servings: 4
Ingredients:

- ½ c. fresh cilantro, chopped

- 1 ¼ tsp. chili powder

- 1 c. fresh tomatoes, diced

- 1 med. yellow onion, diced

- 1 sm. red bell pepper, diced

- 1 tbsp. cumin, ground

- 1 tbsp. extra virgin olive oil

- 1 tbsp. lime juice, fresh

- 1 tsp. dried oregano

- 2 cloves garlic, minced

- 2 lb. celery stalks, diced

- 4 c. chicken broth

- 8 oz. chicken thighs, boneless and skinless, shredded

- 8 oz. cream cheese, softened

Directions:

1. In a pot over medium heat, warm olive oil and, once hot, add celery, red pepper, onion, and garlic and cook it for about 3 minutes or until shiny.

2. Stir the tomatoes into the pot and let cook for another 2 minutes, then add seasonings to the pot, stir in chicken broth and bring to a boil.

3. Once boiling, drop the heat down to low and allow to simmer for 20 minutes.

4. Add the cream cheese and allow the soup to return to a boil, then drop the heat once again and allow to simmer for another 20 minutes.

5. Stir the shredded chicken into the soup along with the lime juice and the cilantro.

6. Spoon into bowls and serve hot!

Nutrition: Calories 420, Fat 29,5, Carbs 9, Protein 29.

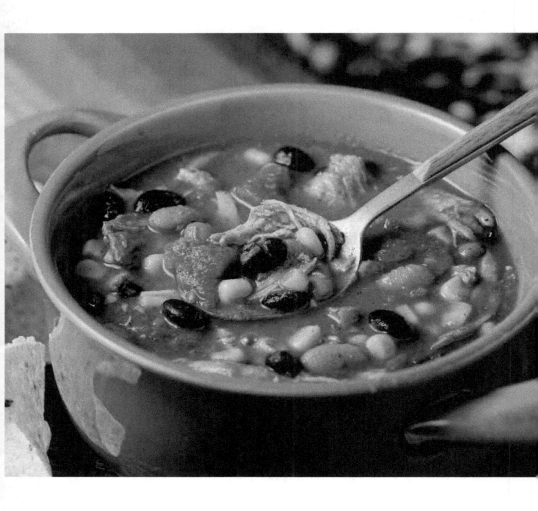

49. Crackpot Chicken Taco Soup

Preparation Time: 15 minutes

Cooking Time: 6 hours

Servings: 6
Ingredients:

- 2 frozen boneless chicken breasts

- 2 cans of white beans or black beans

- 1 can of diced tomatoes

- Green chili's

- ½ onion chopped

- ½ packet of taco seasoning

- ½ teaspoon of Garlic salt

- 1 cup of chicken broth

- Salt and pepper to taste

- Tortilla chips, cheese sour cream, and cilantro as toppings, as well as chili pepper (this is optional).

Directions:

1. Put your frozen chicken with other ingredients into the crockpot and leave to cook for about 6-8 hours.

2. Once it's cooked, take out the chicken and shred it into the size you want.

3. Place the shredded chicken into a slow cooker, stir, and allow to cook.

Note: If you want, you can add more beans and tomatoes also to help stretch the meat and make it tastier.

Nutrition: Calories 492 - Fat 4, Fiber 12, Carbs 47, Protein 29.

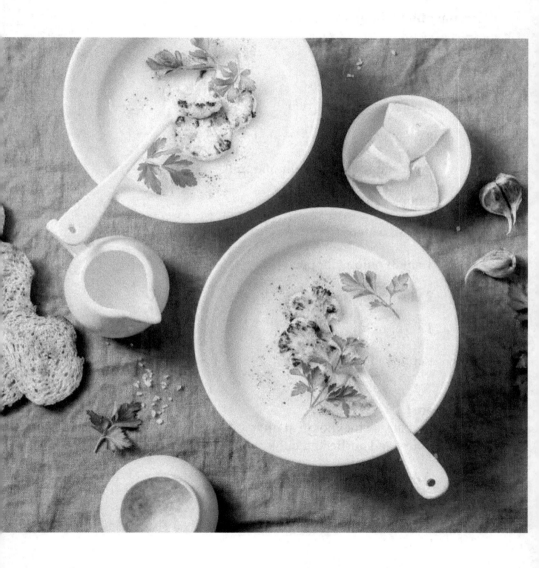

50. Creamy Cauliflower Soup

Preparation Time: 15 minutes

Cooking Time: 30 minutes

Servings: 6

Ingredients:

- 5 cups cauliflower rice

- 8 oz. cheddar cheese, grated

- 2 cups unsweetened almond milk

- 2 cups vegetable stock

- 2 tbsp. water

- 1 small onion, chopped

- 2 garlic cloves, minced

- 1 tbsp. of olive oil

- Pepper and salt

Directions:

1. In a large stockpot heat olive oil over medium heat, then add onion and garlic and cook them for 1-2 minutes.

2. After this, add cauliflower rice and water, cover, and cook for 5-7 minutes.

3. Add vegetable stock and almond milk, stir well, and bring to boil.

4. When it boils, turn heat to low and simmer for 5 minutes.

5. Turn off the heat. Slowly add cheddar cheese and stir until smooth.

6. Finally, season the soup with pepper and salt, stir well and serve hot.

Nutrition: Calories 214, Fat 16,5, Carbs 7,3, Protein 11.

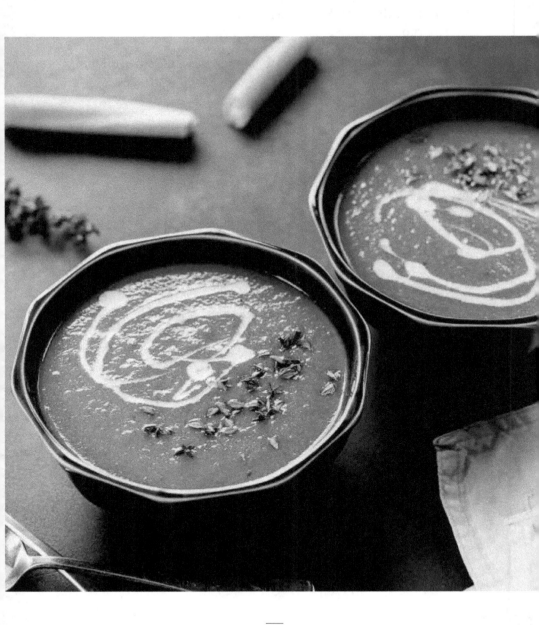

51. Cream of Thyme Tomato Soup

Preparation Time: 5 minutes

Cooking Time: 20 minutes

Servings: 6

Ingredients:

- 2 tbsp. ghee

- 2 large red onions, diced

- ½ cup raw cashew nuts, diced

- 2 (28 oz.) cans tomatoes

- 1 tsp. fresh thyme leaves + extra to garnish

- 1 ½ cups water

- Salt and black pepper to taste

Directions:

1. In a pot, melt ghee over medium heat and sauté the onions for 4 minutes until softened.

2. Stir in the tomatoes, thyme, water, cashews, season with salt and black pepper, cover, and bring to simmer for 10 minutes.

3. Turn the heat off, and puree the ingredients with an immersion blender.

4. Finally, stir in the heavy cream, and serve the soup into soup bowls.

Nutrition: Calories 310, Fat 27, Carbs 3, Protein 11.

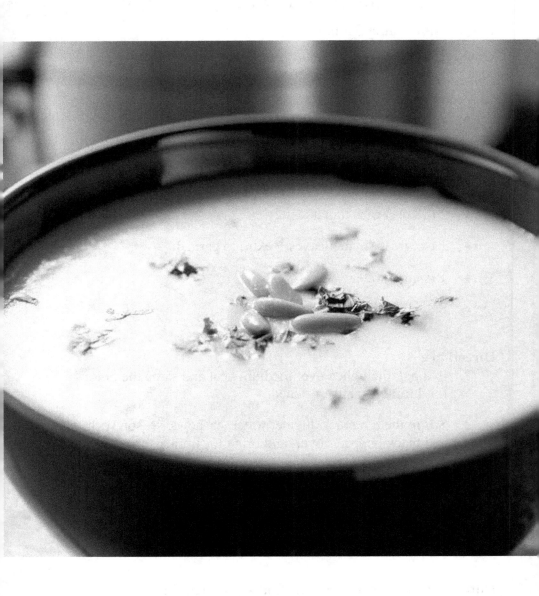

52. Easy Cauliflower Soup

Preparation Time: 5 minutes

Cooking Time: 15 minutes

Servings: 4

Ingredients:

- 2 tbsp of olive oil
- 2 onions, finely chopped
- 1 tsp. garlic, minced
- 1-pound cauliflower, cut into florets
- 1 cup of kale, chopped
- 4 cups of vegetable broth
- ½ cup of almond milk
- ½ tsp. of salt
- ½ tsp. red pepper flakes
- 1 tbsp. fresh chopped parsley

Directions:

1. In a pot, warm the oil over medium heat, then add garlic and onions and sauté until browned and softened.

2. Place in the pot the vegetable broth, kale, and cauliflower and cook for 10 minutes until the mixture boils.

3. When it boils, stir in the pepper flakes, salt, and almond milk, reduce the heat and simmer the soup for 5 minutes.

4. Transfer the soup to an immersion blender and blend to achieve the desired consistency.

5. Finally, top with parsley and serve immediately.

Nutrition: Calories 172, Fat 10,3, Carbs 1,8, Protein 8,1.

53. Healthy Chicken Taco Soup

Preparation Time: 5 minutes

Cooking Time: 20 minutes

Servings: 8-10

Ingredients:
- ½ tbsp avocado or coconut oil
- 1 small yellow onion, diced
- 1 small red bell pepper, diced
- 1 small green bell pepper, diced
- 5 cloves garlic, minced
- 1 lb boneless, skinless chicken breast
- 1 ½ tsp salt (plus more to taste)
- 1 tsp dried oregano
- 1 tsp chipotle powder
- 1 tsp paprika
- 2 tsp cumin
- ¼ tsp black pepper
- 1 – 15 oz can fire roasted diced tomatoes
- 2 – 4.5 oz cans green chilies
- ¼ c. fresh lime juice
- 32 oz chicken broth
- Cilantro, for serving
- Diced red onion, for serving
- Lime wedges, for serving

Directions:
1. Heat a large pot over medium-high heat and once hot, add in the avocado (or coconut oil), the peppers, onion, and garlic and saute for 3-4 minutes until the onions start to become translucent.

2. Add the chicken breast, canned tomatoes, canned green chilies, spices, lime juice, and chicken broth to the pot and stir until well combined.

3. When it boil, reduce the heat to a simmer and allow the soup to simmer for 30 minutes.

4. Transfer the chicken breast to a small bowl and use two forks to shred the meat.

5. Add the chicken back to the soup and stir until well combined.

6. Finally, serve the soup with fresh cilantro, diced red onion, and fresh lime wedges.

Nutrition: Calories 258, Fat 6,1, Fiber 5,1, Carbs 22,7, Protein 30.

54. Lime-Mint Soup

Preparation Time: 5 minutes

Cooking Time: 20 minutes

Servings: 4

Ingredients:

- 4 cups vegetable broth

- ¼ cup fresh mint leaves, roughly chopped

- ¼ cup chopped scallions, white and green parts

- 3 garlic cloves, minced

- 3 tablespoons freshly squeezed lime juice

Directions:

1. In a large stockpot, combine the broth, mint, scallions, garlic, and lime juice and bring to a boil over medium-high heat.

2. Reduce the heat to low, simmer for 15 minutes, and serve.

Nutrition: Calories 6, Fat 0, Fiber 0,2, Carbs 1,4, Protein 0,1.

55. Quick Lentil Chili

Preparation Time: 15 minutes

Cooking Time: 1 hour 20 minutes

Servings: 10
Ingredients:
- 1 ½ cups of seeded or diced pepper
- 1 ½ cups of coarsely chopped onions
- 5 cups of vegetable broth (it should have a low sodium content)
- 1 tablespoon of garlic
- ¼ teaspoon of freshly ground pepper
- 1 cup of red lentils
- 3 filled teaspoons of chili powder
- 1 tablespoon of grounded cumin

Directions:
1. In a pot, combine the onions, red peppers, low sodium vegetable broth, garlic, salt, and pepper and cook them over medium heat.

2. Cook for about 10 minutes and stir frequently until the onions are more translucent, and all the liquid evaporated.

3. Then, add the remaining broth, lime juice, chili powder, lentils, cumin, and boil.

4. Then, reduce heat and cook for about 1 hour to a simmer until the lentils are appropriately cooked (if the mixture seems to be thick, add a little water).

5. The chili will be appropriately done when most of the water is absorbed. Once it's cooked, serve hot and enjoy!

Note: Store the lentil chili in a sealed container in the fridge for up to 5 days.

Nutrition: Calories 112,5 - Fat 2,9, Fiber 3,3, Carbs 12,1, Protein 2,3.

56.   Roasted Tomato Soup

Preparation Time: 20 minutes

Cooking Time: 50 minutes

Servings: 6

Ingredients:

- 3 pounds of tomatoes (halved)

- 6 garlic (smashed)

- 2 onions (cut)

- 4 teaspoon of cooking oil or virgin oil

- Salt to taste

- Freshly grounds pepper

- ¼ cup of heavy cream

- Sliced fresh basil leaves for garnish

Directions:

1. Preheat the oven to 427 °F and prepare a baking sheet.

2. Into a bowl, mix the halved tomatoes, garlic, olive oil, onions, salt, and pepper, and spread the tomato mixture on the baking sheet.

3. Roast for about 20-28 minutes stirring from time to time.

4. Remove it from the oven, and transfer the roasted vegetables to a soup pot.

5. Add in the pot the basil leaves and blend in small portions in a blender. Then serve immediately.

Nutrition: Calories 142,5 - Fat 5,9, Carbs 12,6, Protein 2,3.

57.   Slow Cooker Taco Soup

Preparation Time: 10 minutes

Cooking Time: 2 hours

Servings: 8
Ingredients:

- ¼ c. sour cream

- ½ c. cheddar cheese, shredded

- 2 c. diced tomatoes

- 2 lbs. ground beef

- 3 tbsp. taco seasoning (without hidden sugars or starches).

- 4 c. chicken broth

- 8 oz. cream cheese, cubed

Directions:
1. Heat a medium saucepan over medium heat and brown the beef.

2. Drain the fat from the beef and then place it into the slow cooker with the cream cheese cubes, taco seasoning, and diced tomatoes.

3. Add the chicken broth, cover, and leave to cook on medium heat for two hours.

4. Finally, stir all the ingredients, spoon the soup into bowls and serve hot with sour cream and shredded cheese on top! Enjoy!

Nutrition: Calories 305, Fat 31,5, Carbs 8,5, Protein 43,5.

CPSIA information can be obtained
at www.ICGtesting.com
Printed in the USA
BVHW040241270621
610451BV00005B/1142